Devlin's Heart

Sheila Johnson

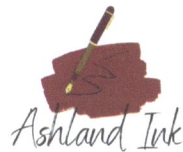

Ashland Ink

About Devlin and this Story

This story is about a real little girl named Devlin who makes the world a much happier place. When she was a baby, Devlin had surgery on her heart. Her family is in awe of her bravery every day.

Devlin's Grammy, Sheila, wrote this story in honor of her granddaughter's courage and strength and to encourage kids everywhere to be brave during life's challenges.

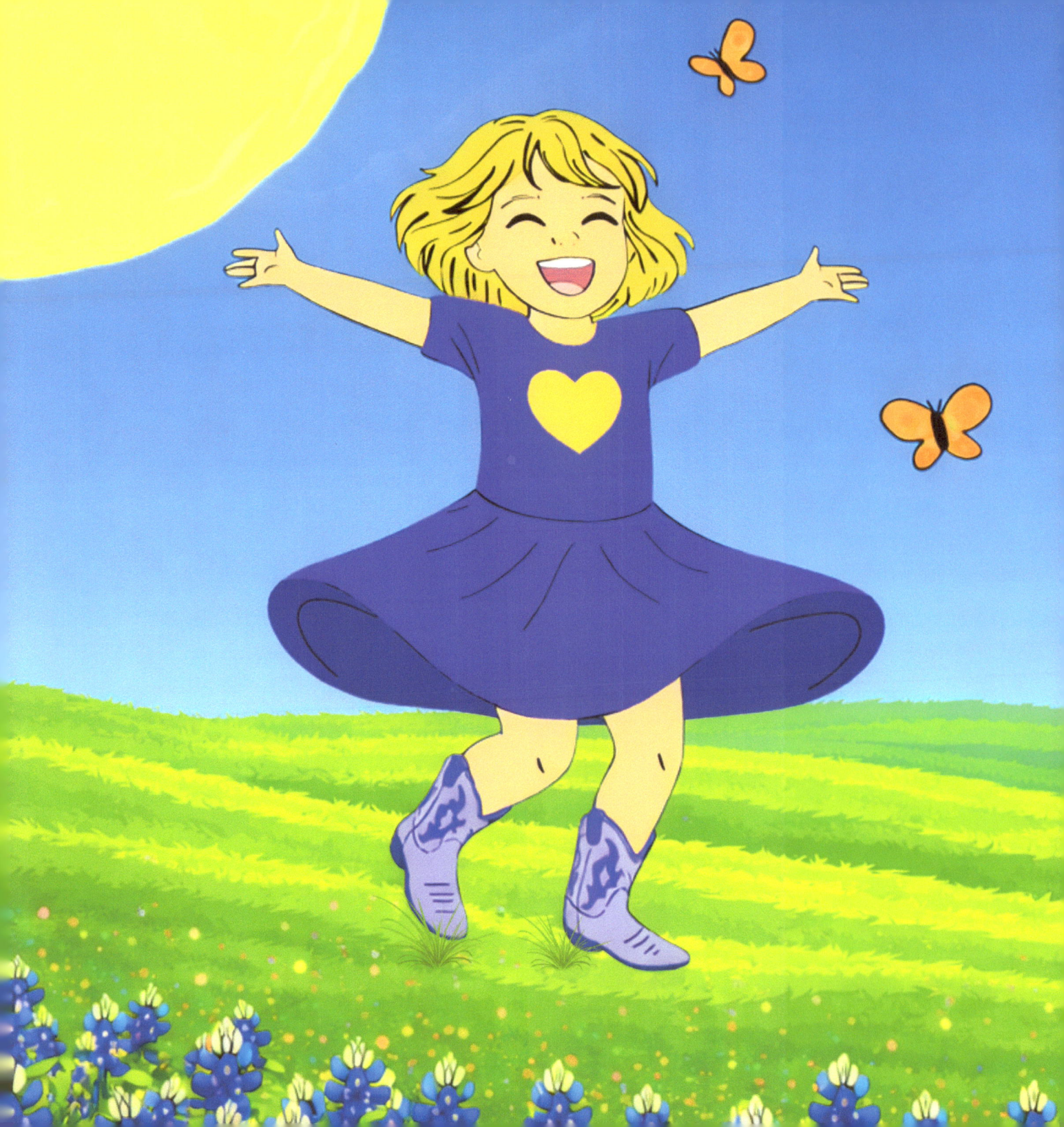

Devlin was a little girl with a smile as warm as sunshine. She giggled, she wiggled, and she looked at the world with big, curious eyes. Everyone who met her said the same thing...

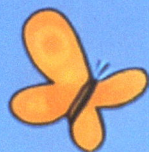

"THAT GIRL IS A FIGHTER!"

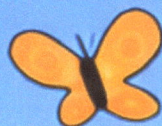

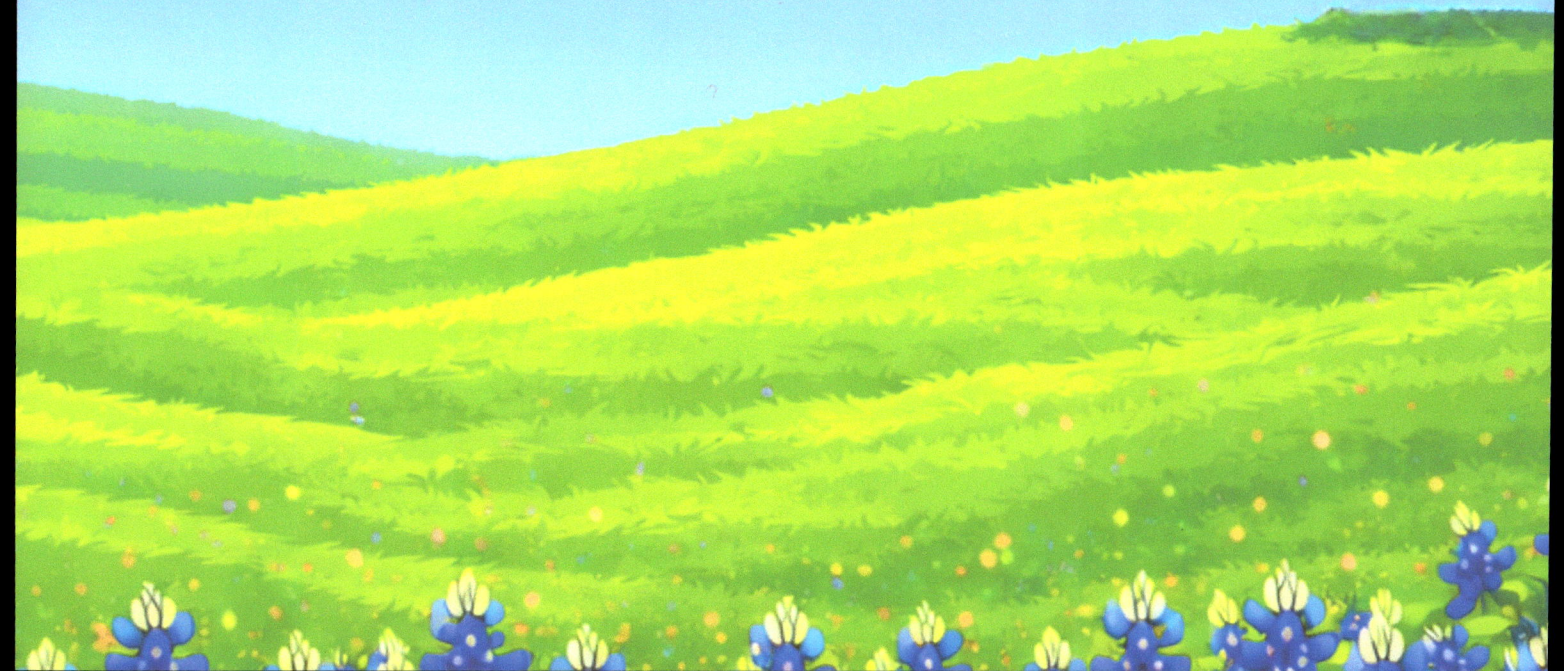

Before she was even born, Mom and Dad hoped and prayed for her.

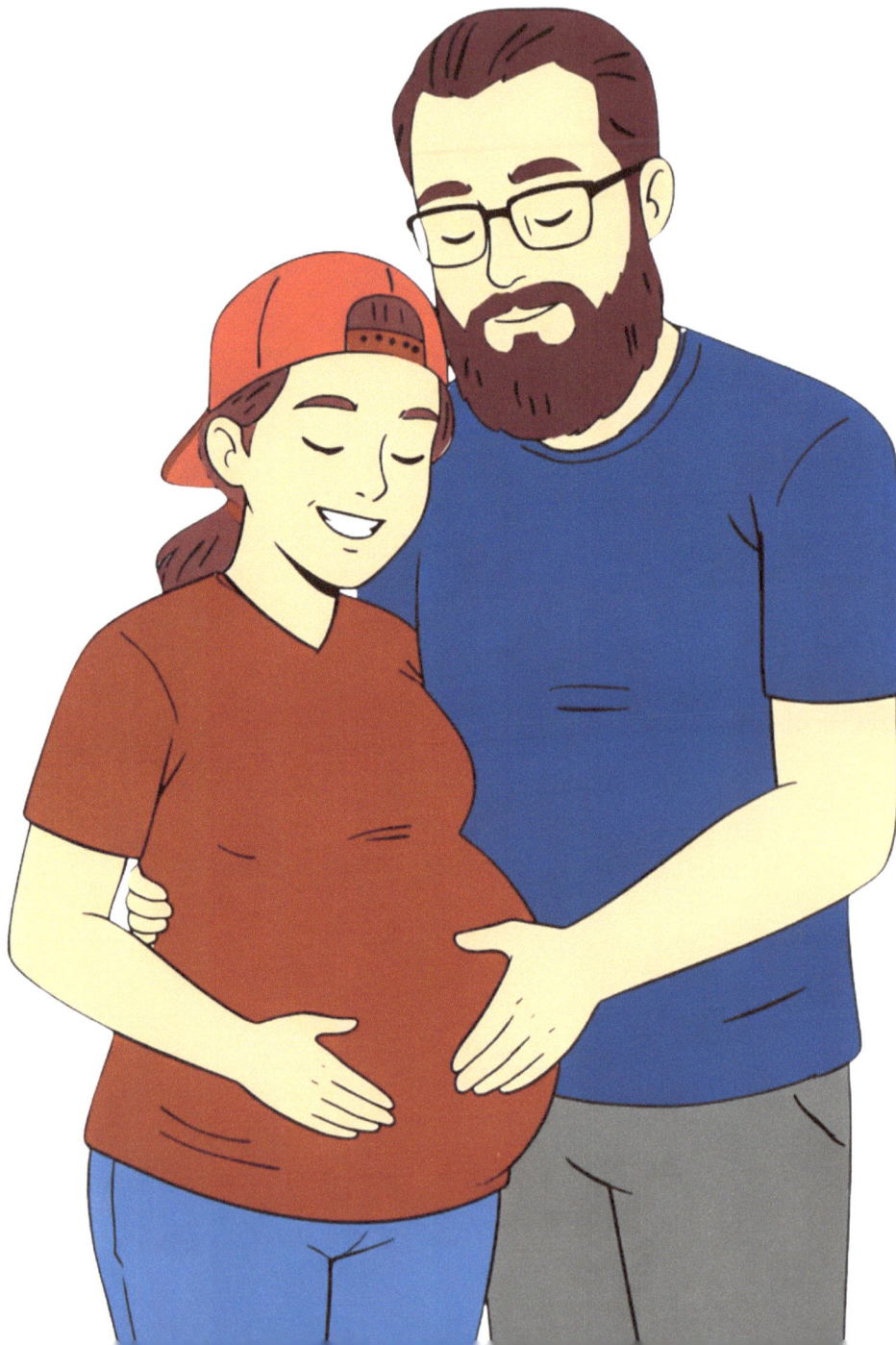

Mom had some hard days during the pregnancy, and the doctors watched Devlin's tiny heart very carefully.

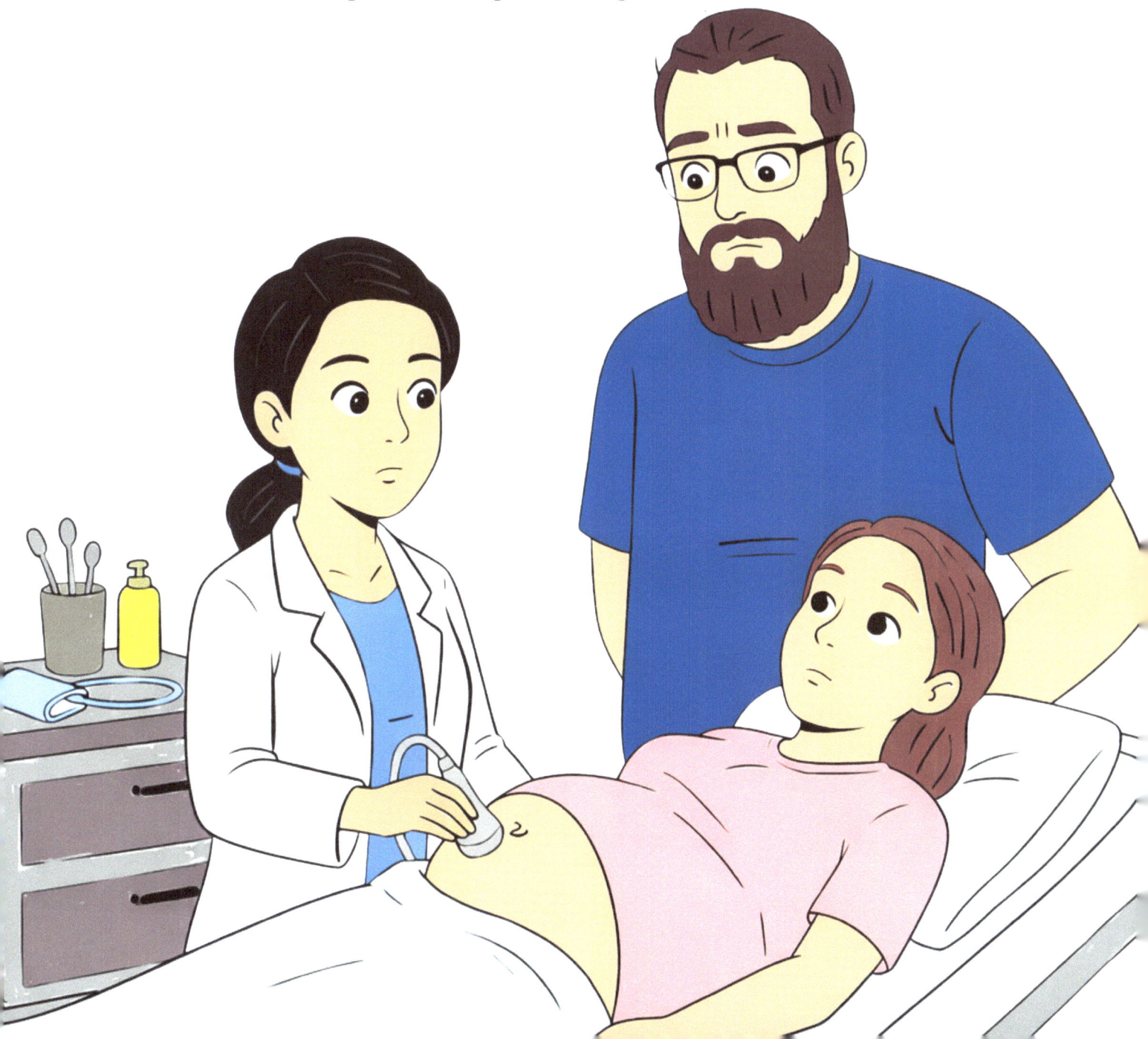

But when Devlin arrived... **oh my!**

She surprised everyone by being strong, sweet, and full of joy.

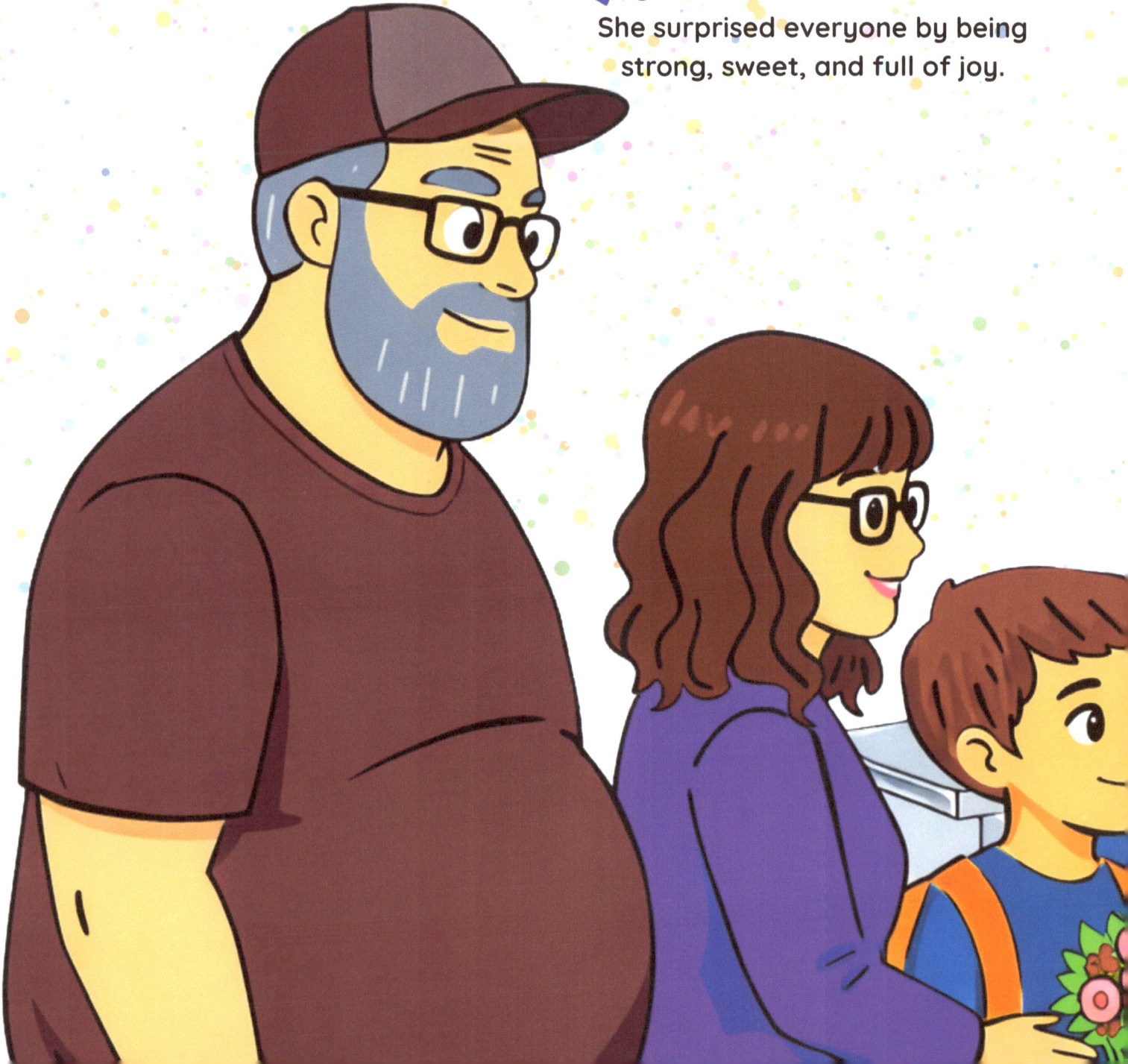

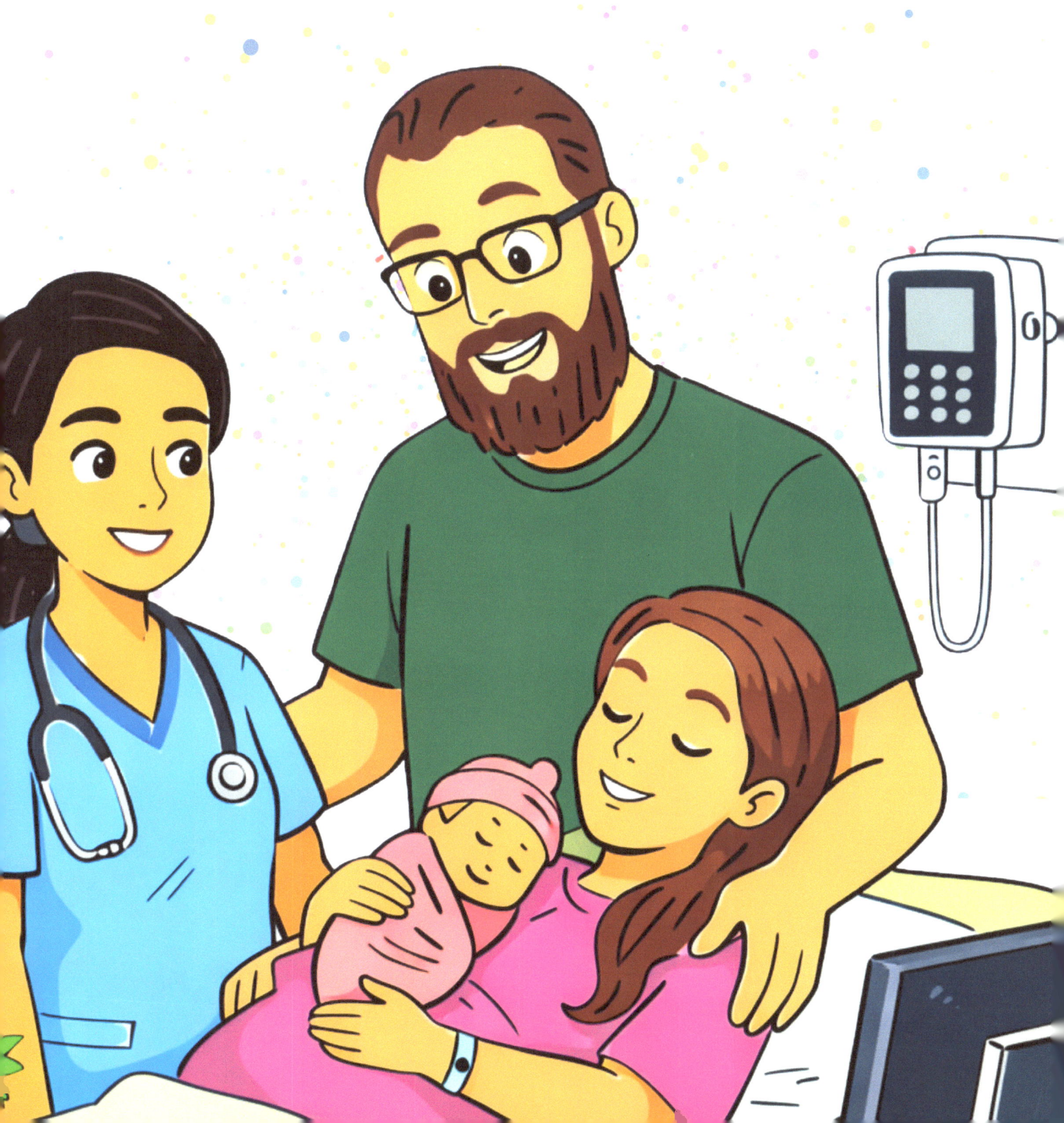

Devlin loved to smile and coo and reach for the
people who loved her most.

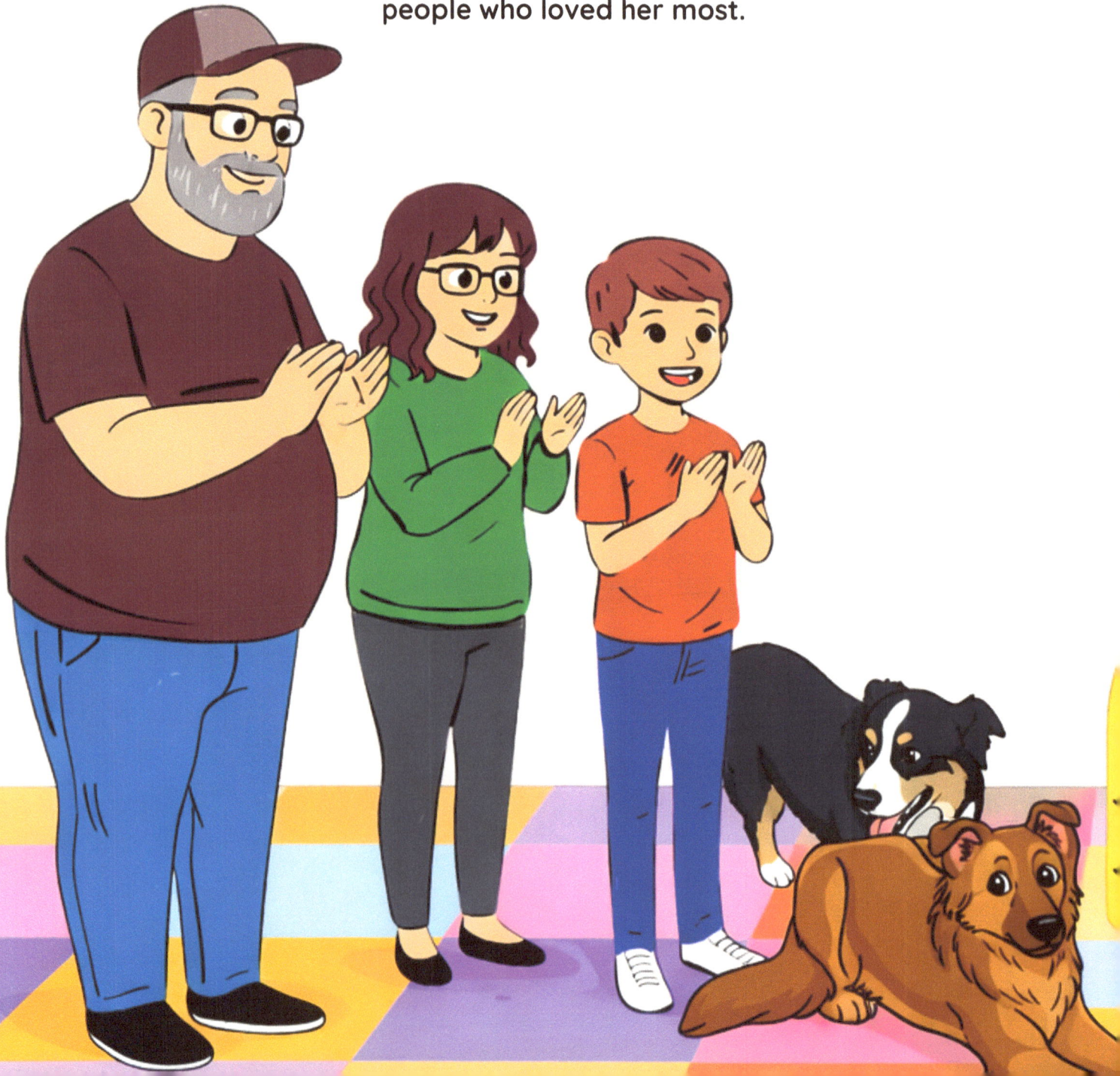

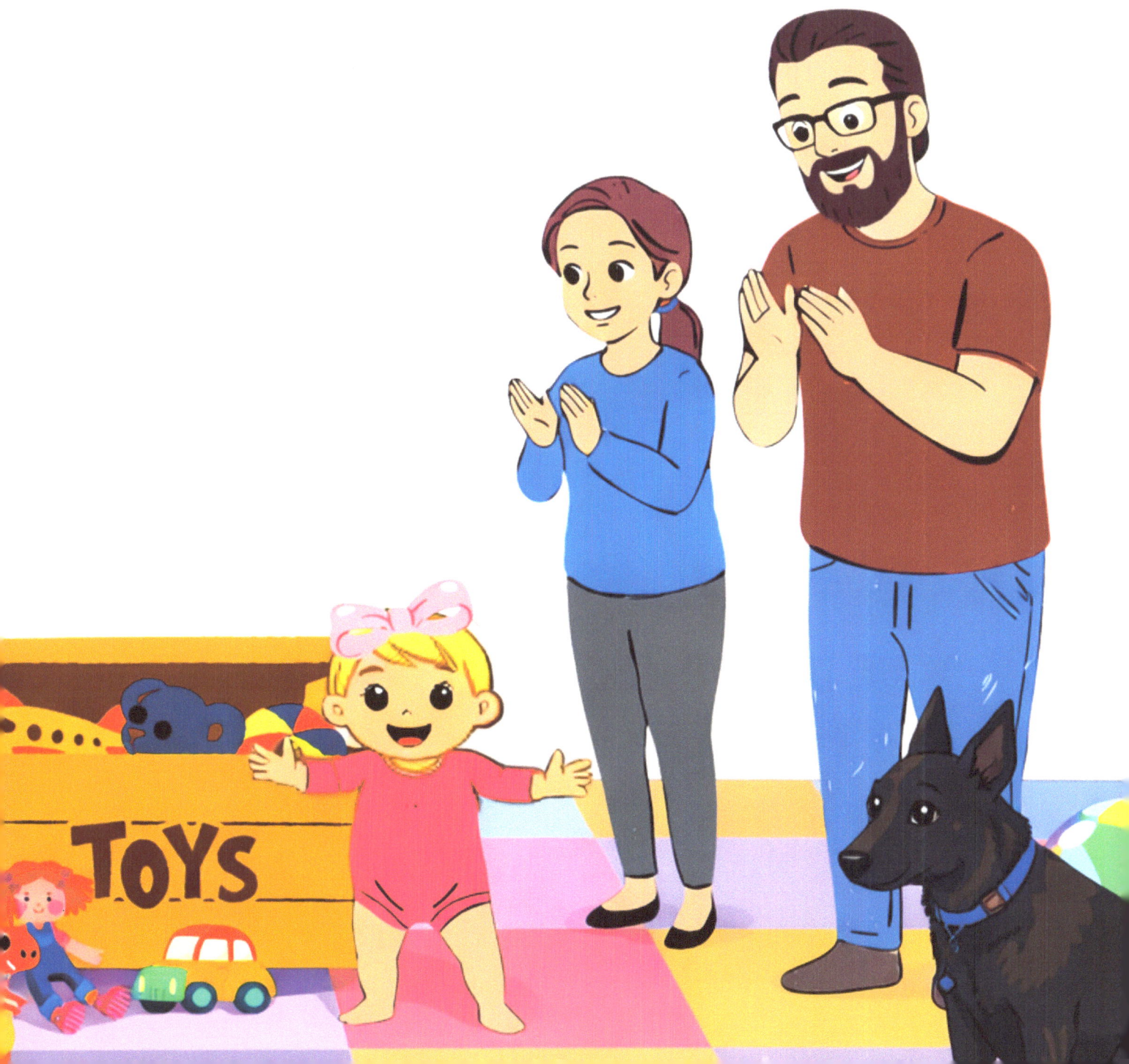

TOYS

But Devlin had a little hole in her heart that needed fixing. So when she was nine months old, Mom, Dad, and the whole family gathered close.

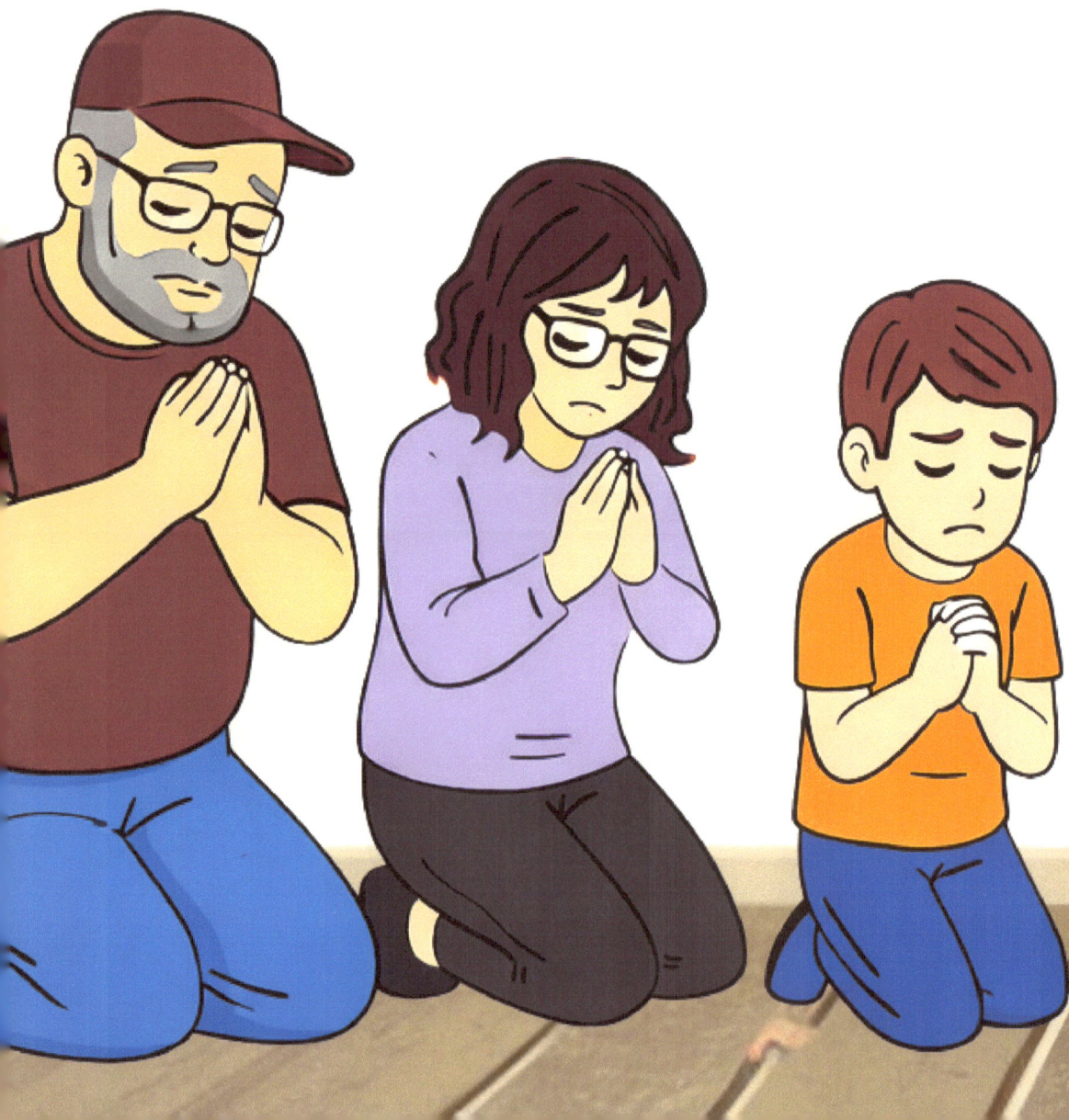

They whispered prayers and trusted
the doctors who were ready to help.

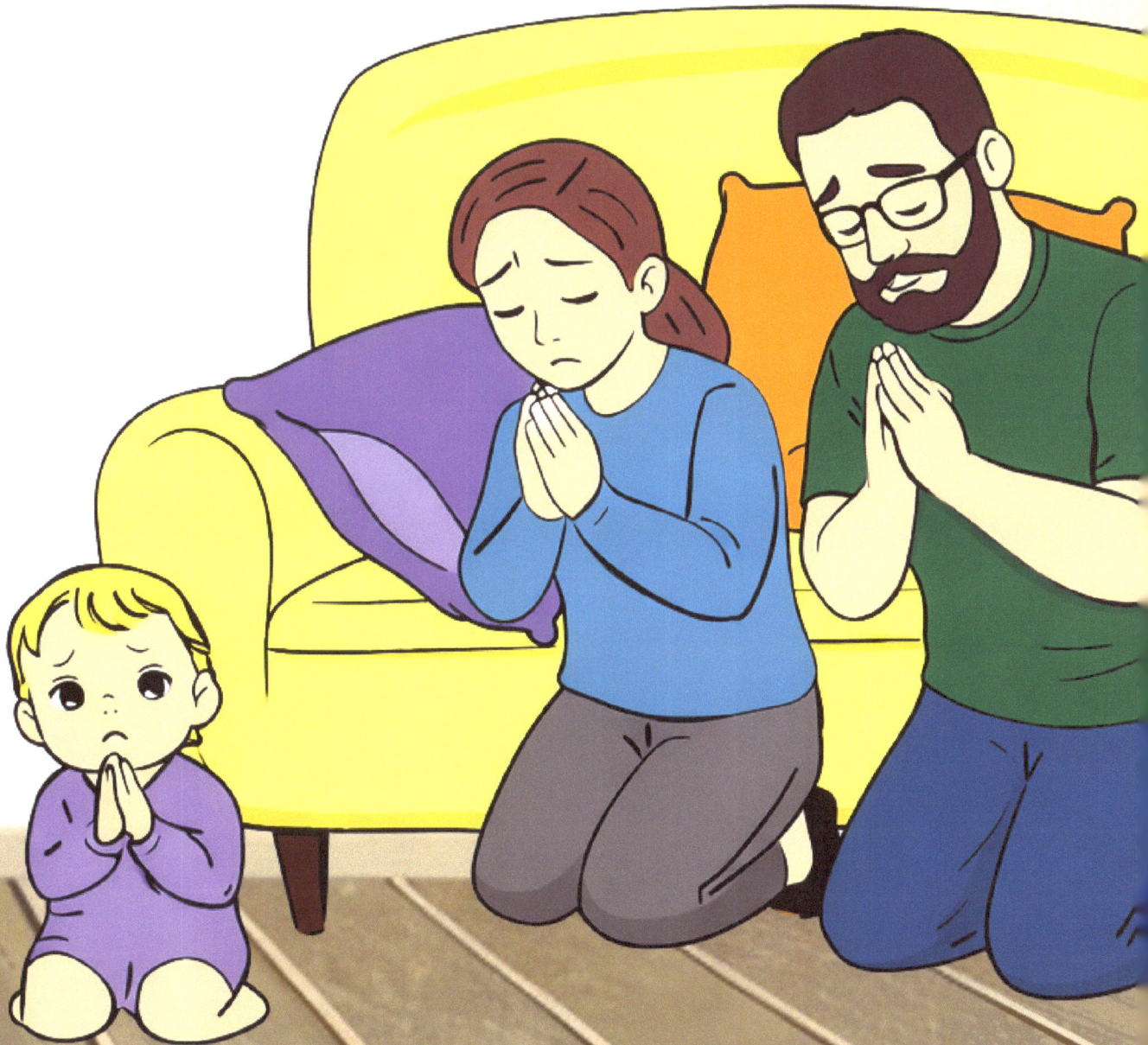

The doctors worked carefully and gently. And when they were done, they said the words everyone had been waiting for...

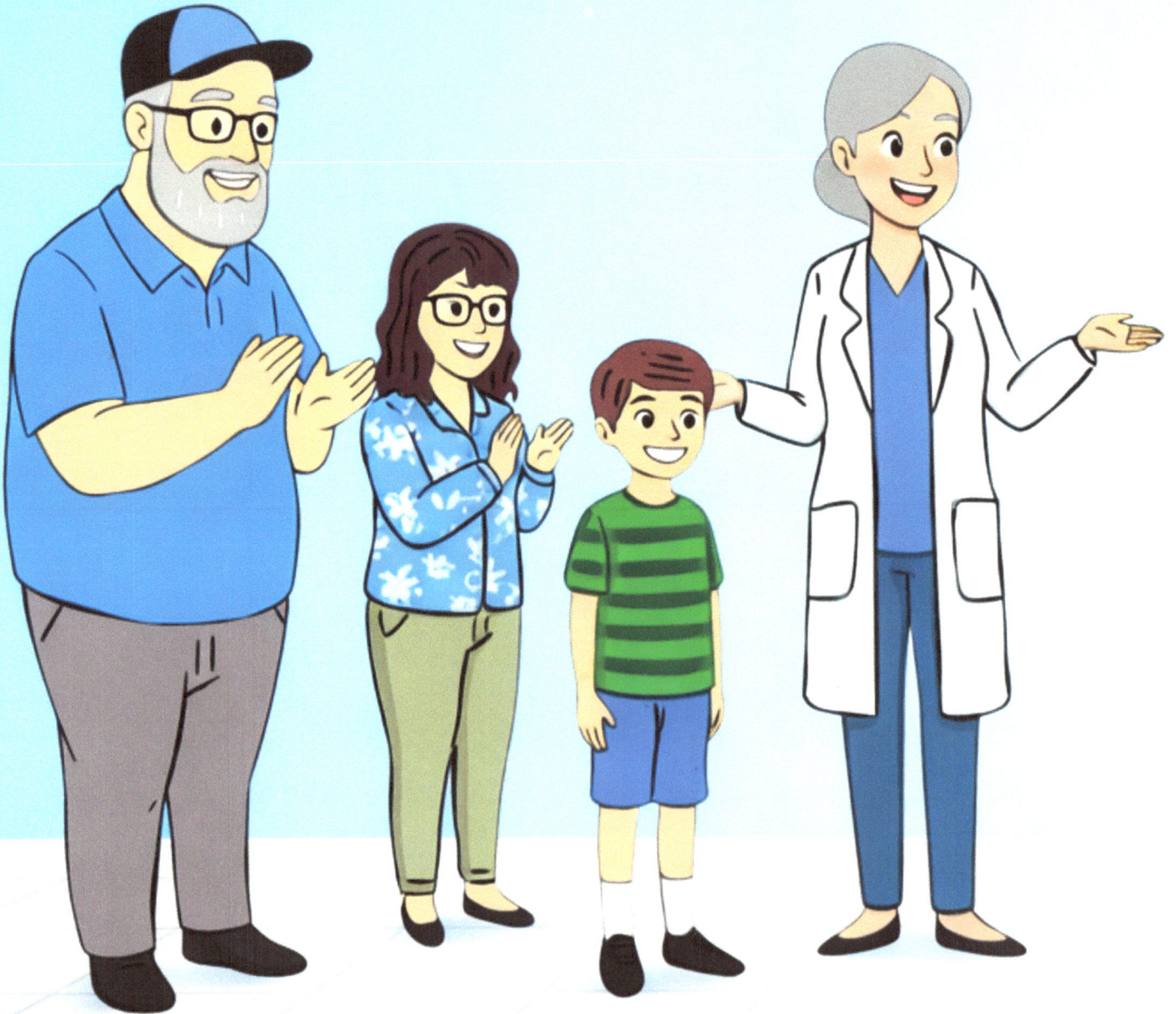

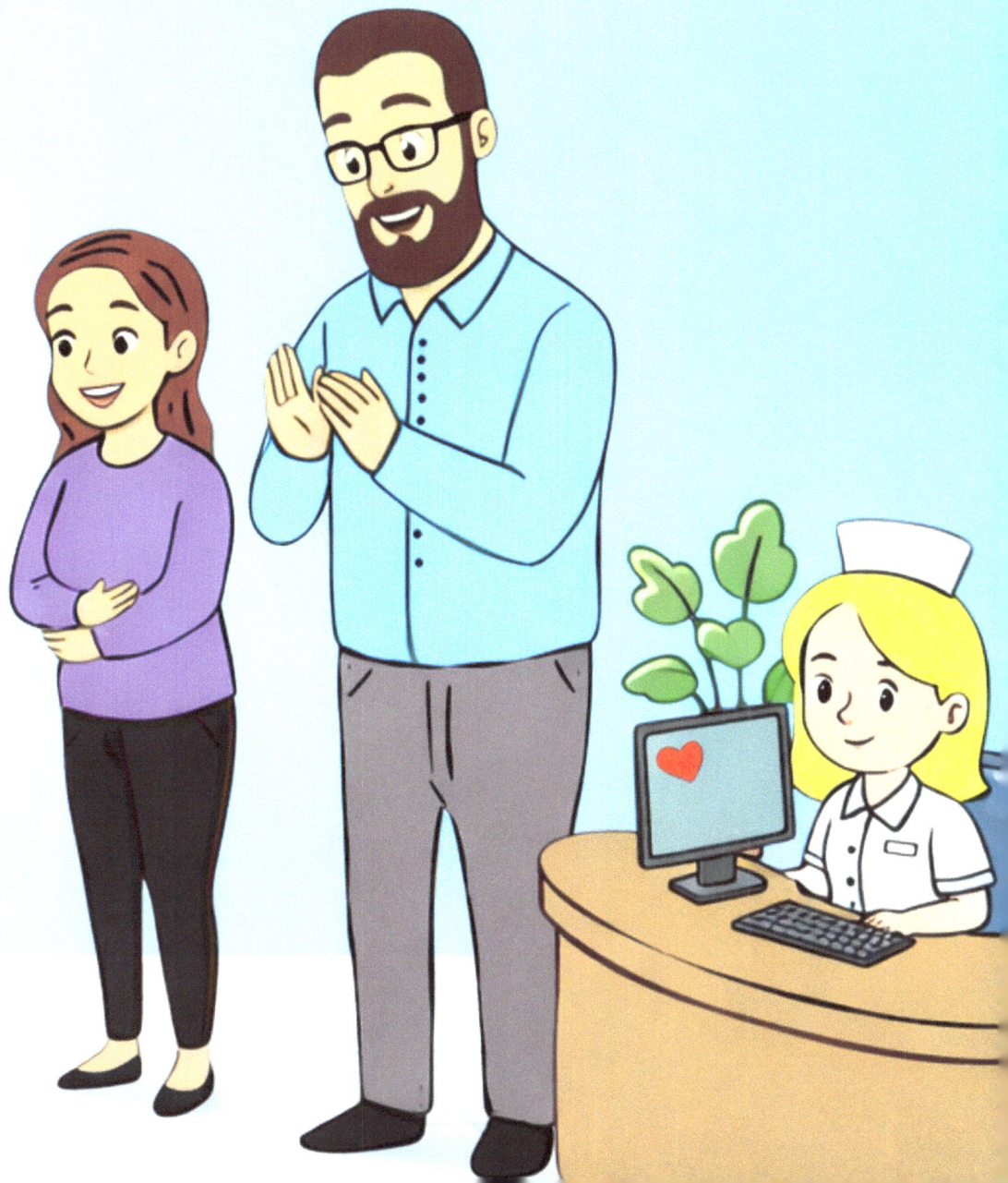

"DEVLIN'S HEART IS REPAIRED!"

In the hospital, Devlin didn't want to stay still for long. Even with wires and monitors, she was soon toddling around in her little gown, pushing her walker and charming the nurses.
"Slow down, sweetheart!" they laughed.

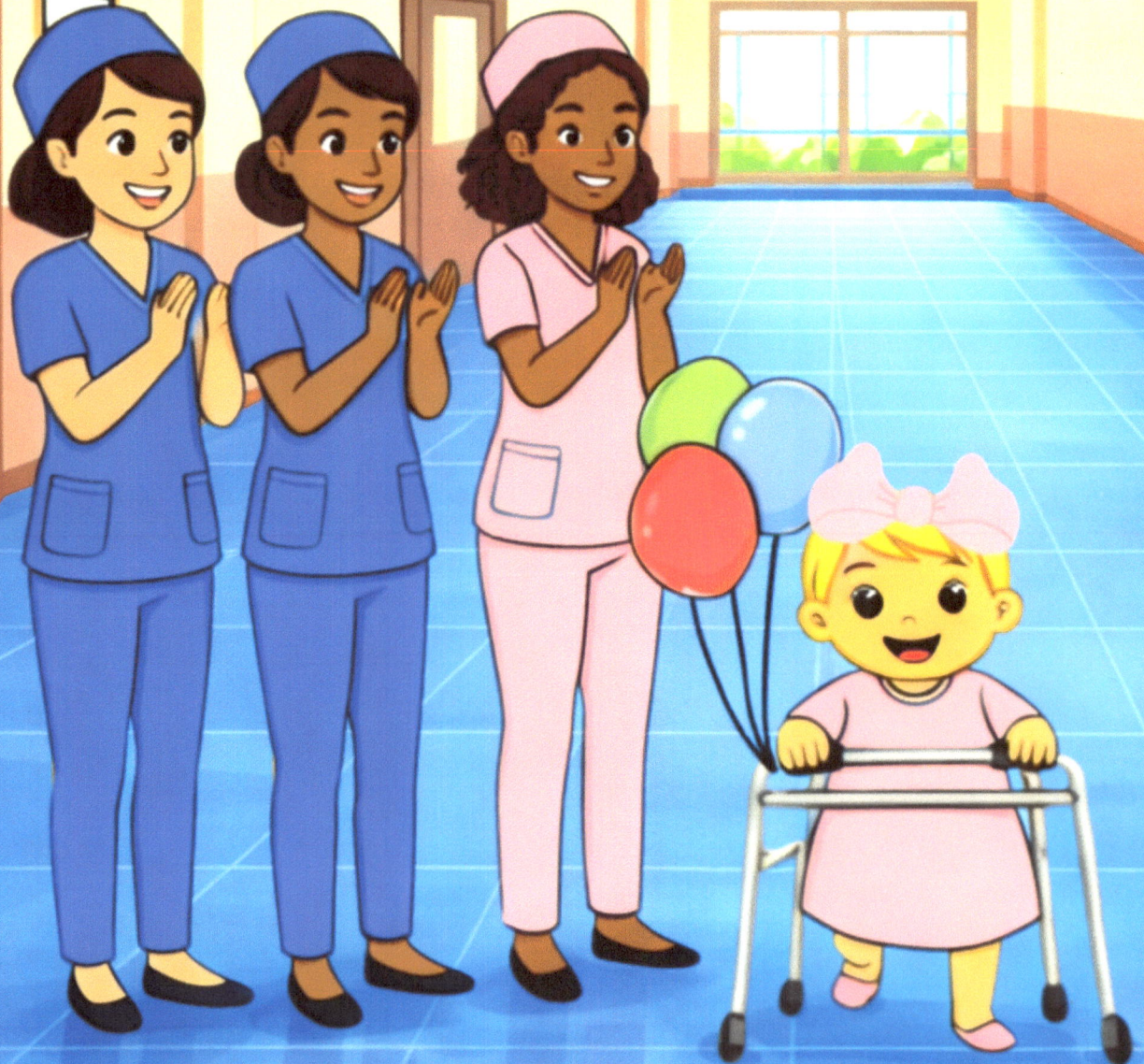

But Devlin was already on the move, ready to go home and ready to grow strong.

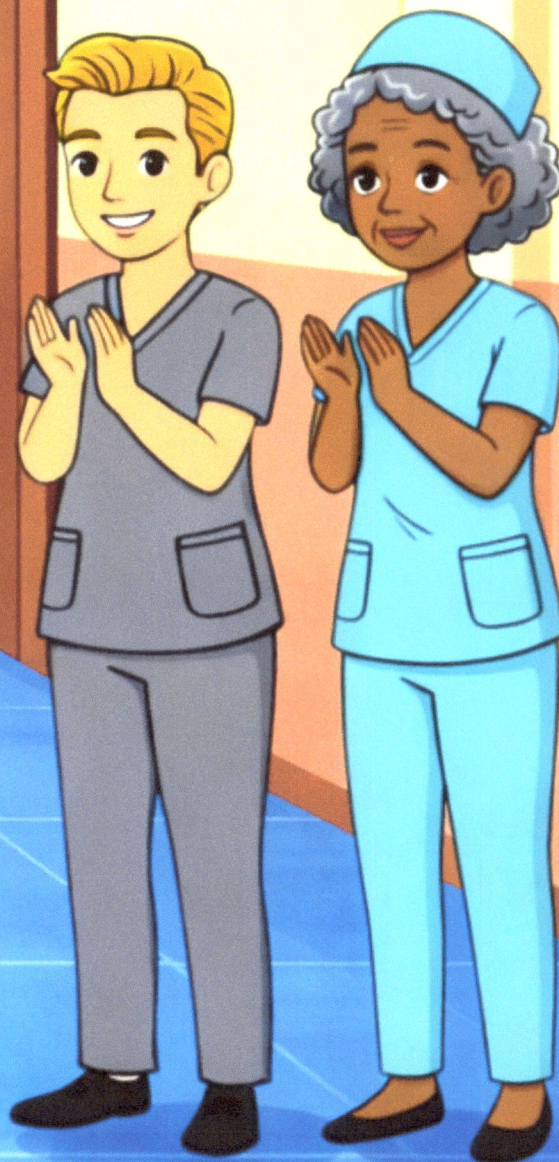

Her heart worked so hard to heal. But sometimes Devlin still got very sick, and she had to visit the hospital again. Whenever she did, her family wrapped her in love and prayers.

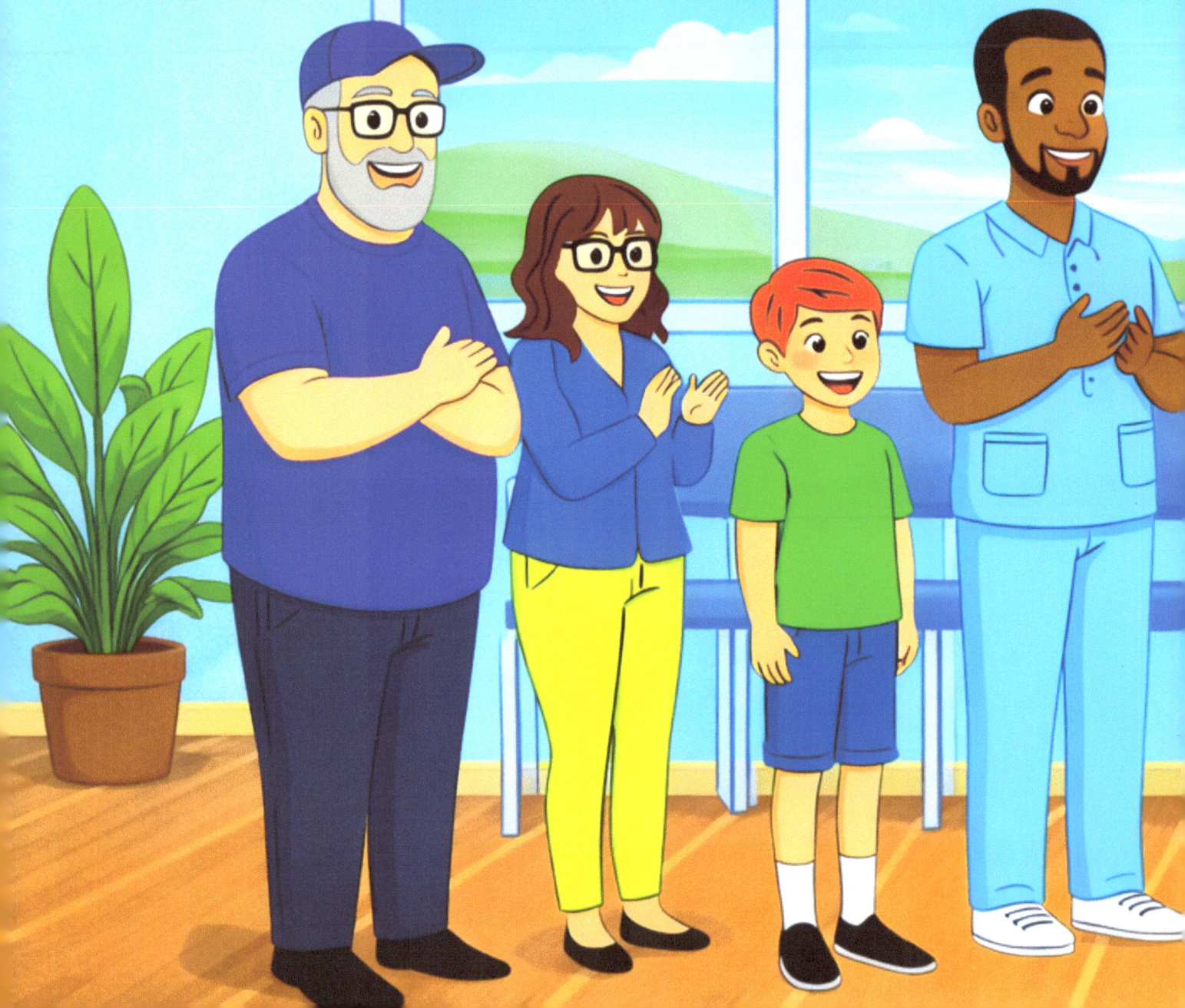

And every time, Devlin showed them just how brave she could be.

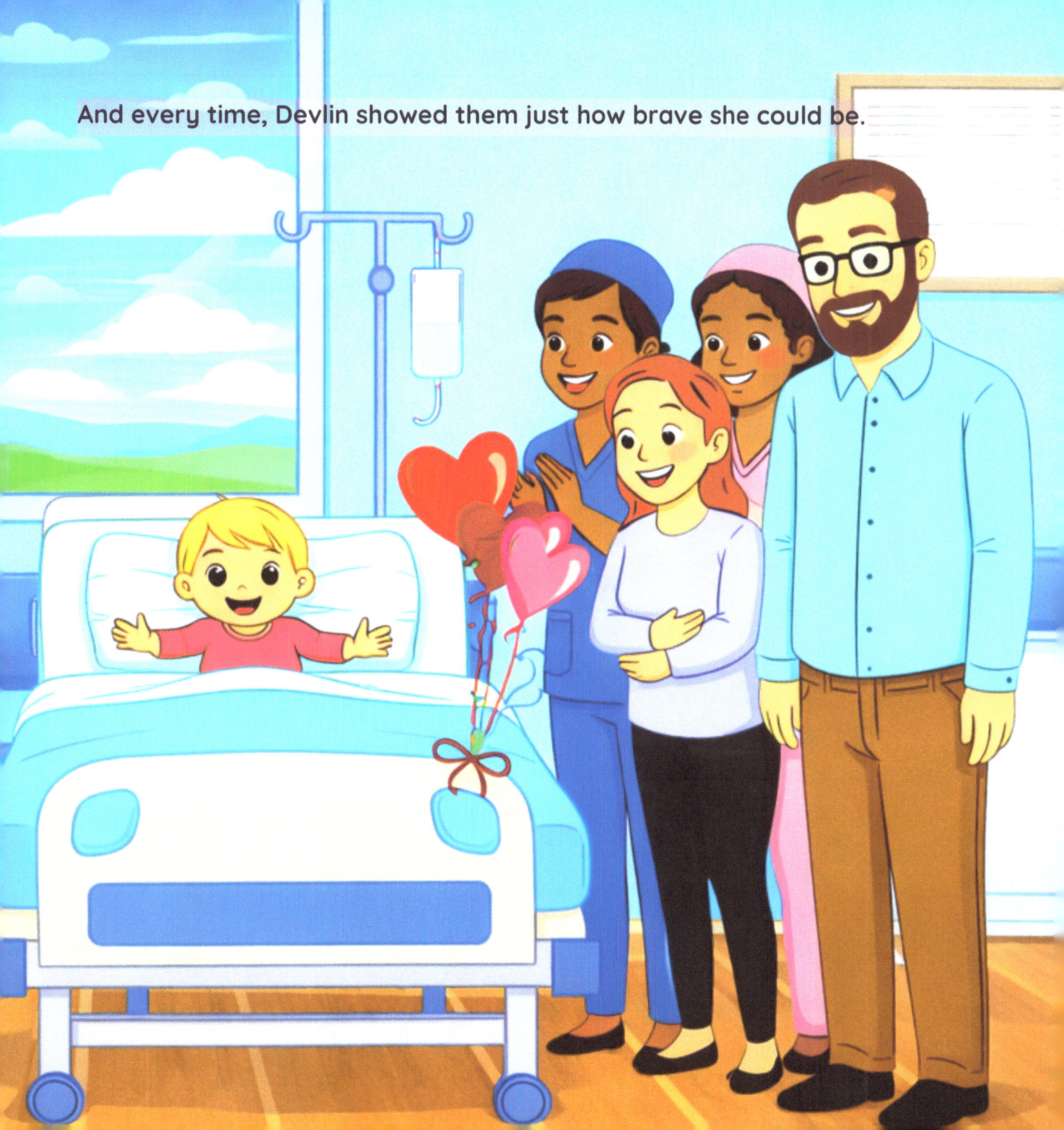

Day by day, Devlin grew stronger. Her smile came back brighter than ever, the kind that can light up a whole room.

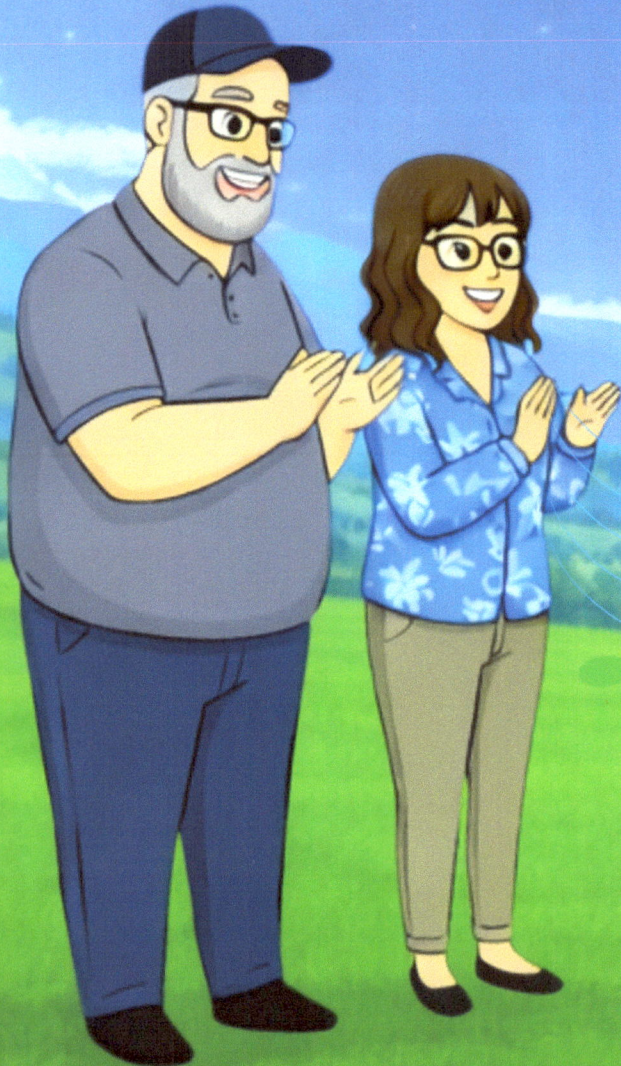

Her laugh bubbled out like music, making everyone around her laugh too.

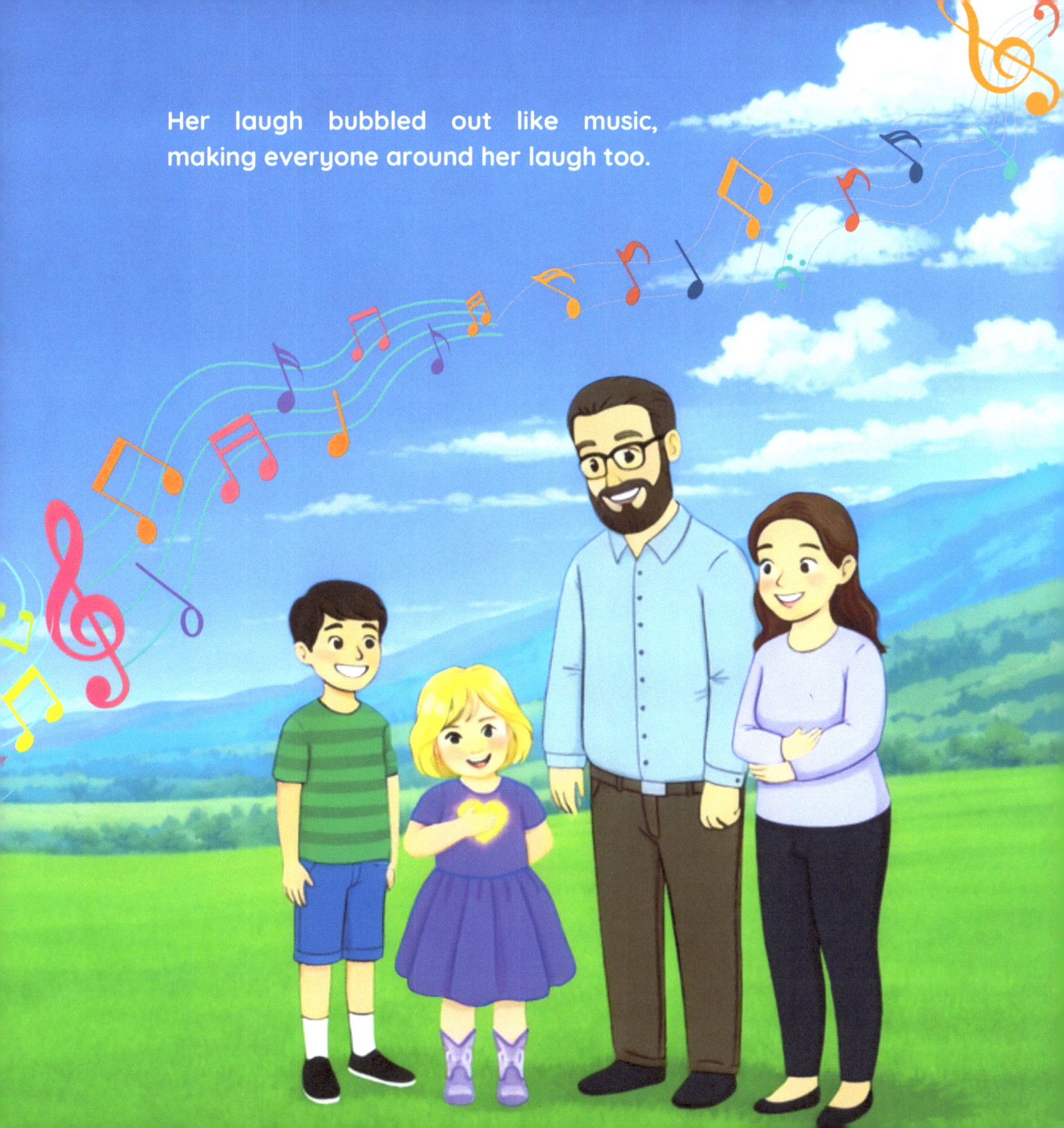

Devlin loved the simple, wonderful things that made her world happy...

Her baby dolls... she dressed them, tucked them in, and pushed them in their little stroller.

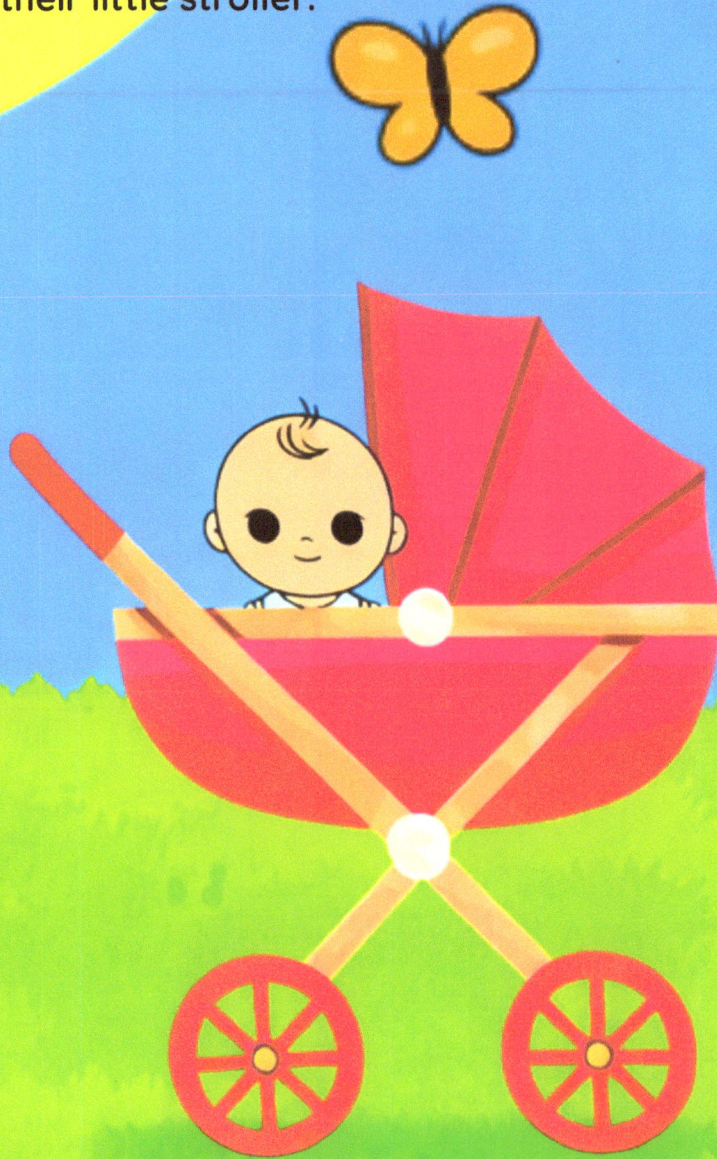

Her puppies... they wagged and wiggled the moment they saw her.
And her playhouse at Grammy and Papa's... her favorite place of all.

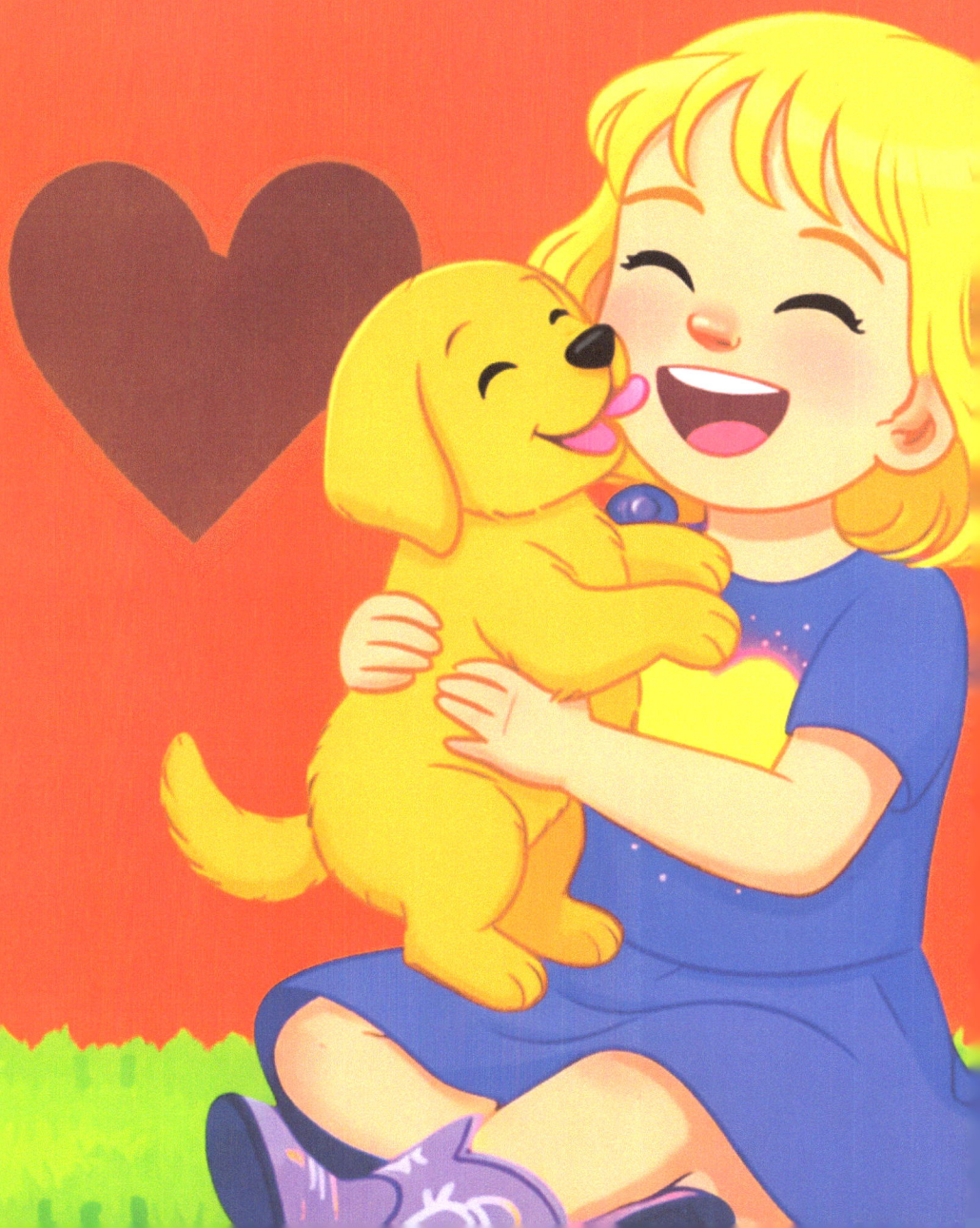

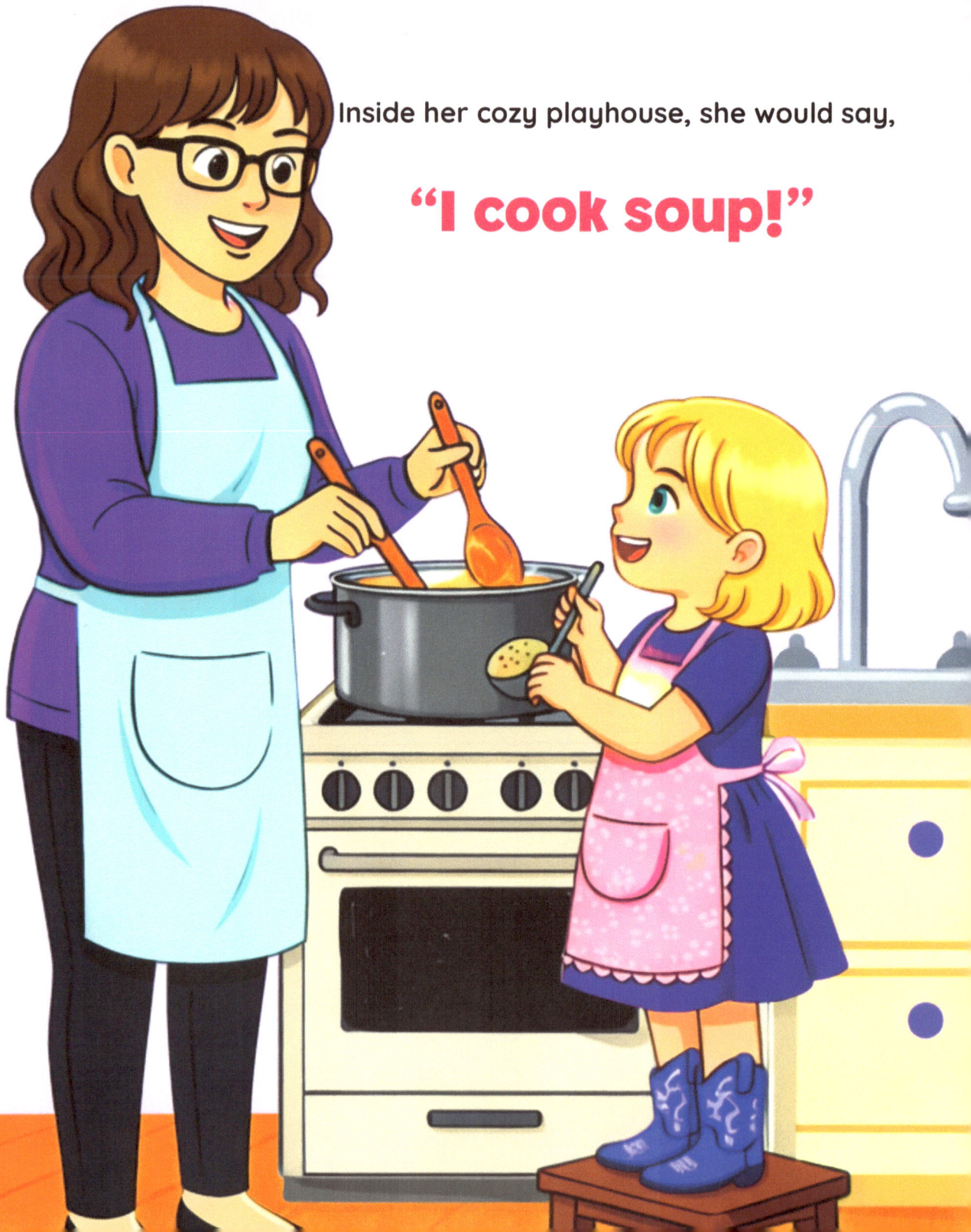

Inside her cozy playhouse, she would say,

"I cook soup!"

She stirred pretend pots, washed her dishes (sometimes using real water!), and kept everything neat and tidy, just like Grammy.

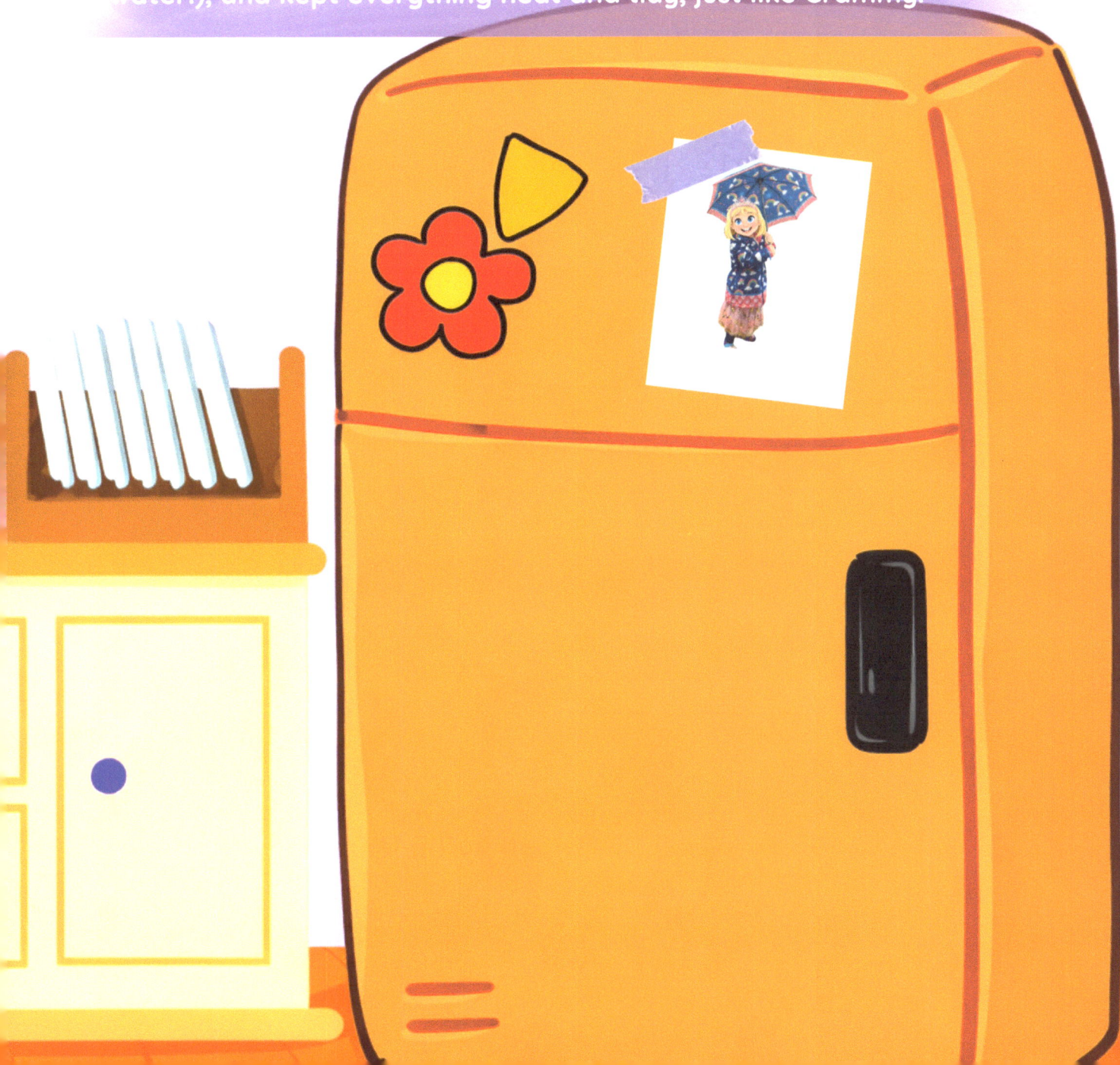

Everyone who knows Devlin sees the same thing...
a strong, joyful girl with a brave heart, a heart that keeps growing
and shining every single day.

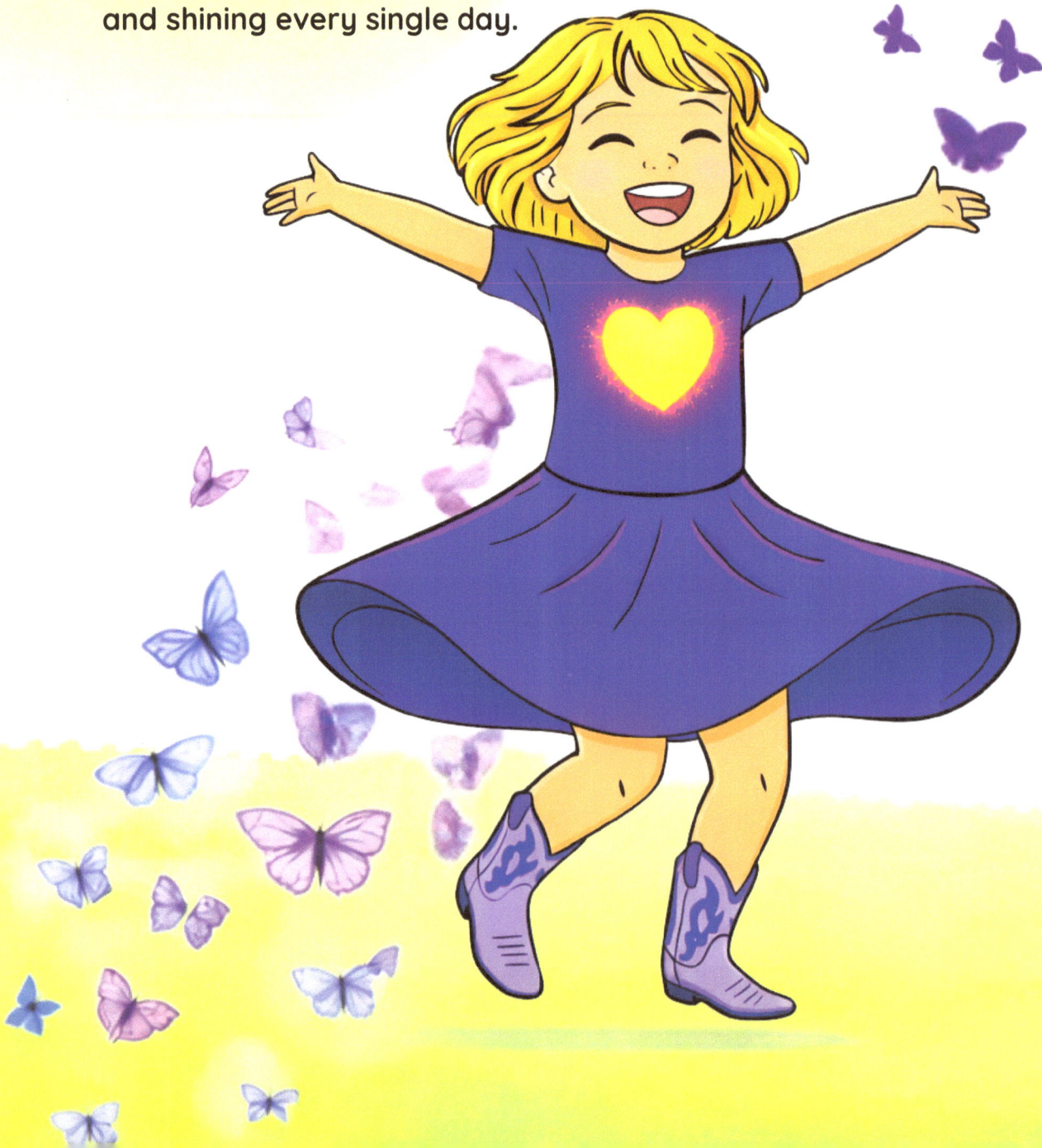

And every day, Devlin shows the world that she is more than a fighter.

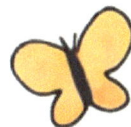

SHE IS LAUGHTER.
SHE IS LIGHT.
SHE IS LOVE.
SHE IS DEVLIN.

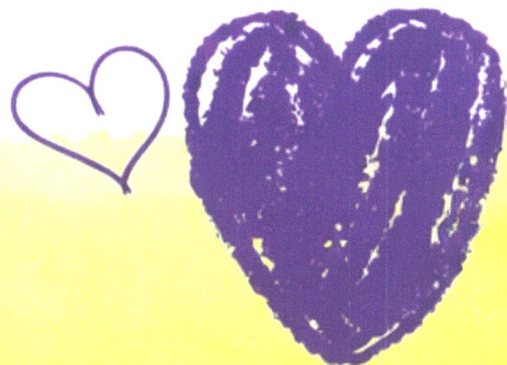

Devlin's Heart is ready to take on the World!

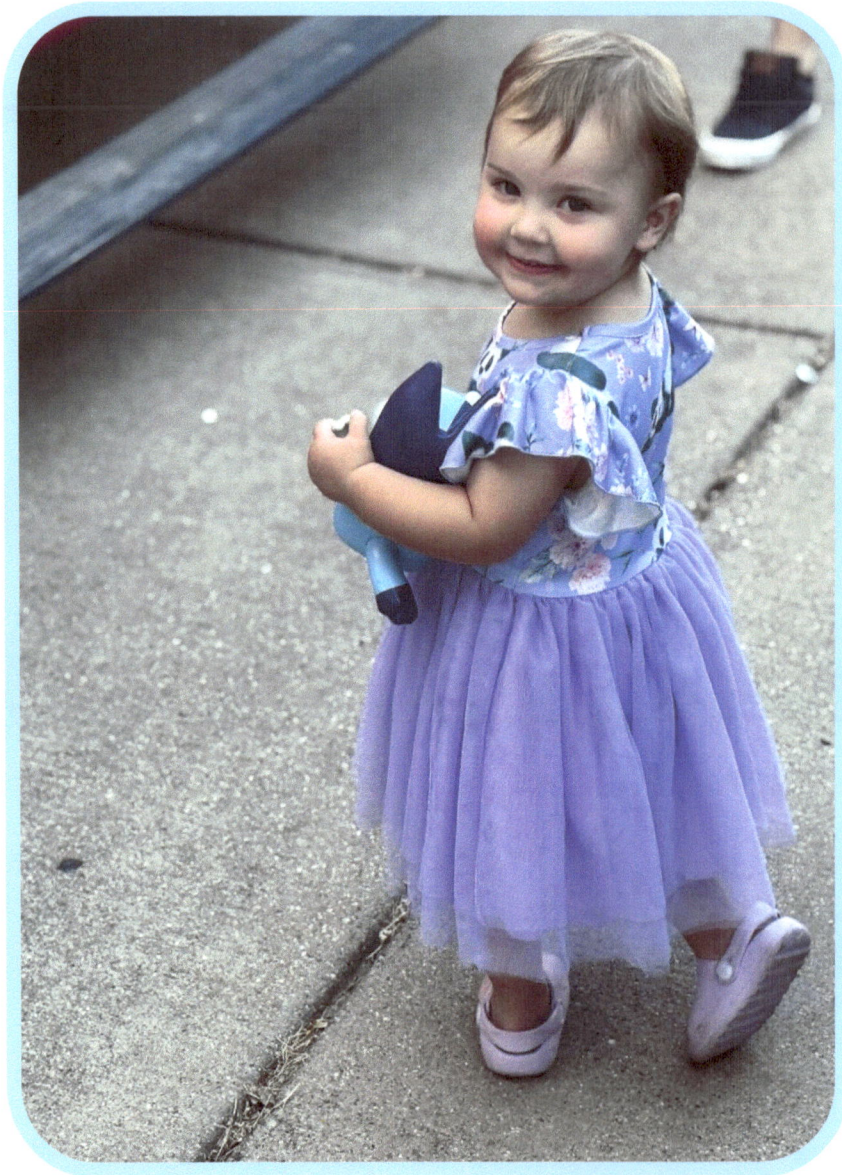

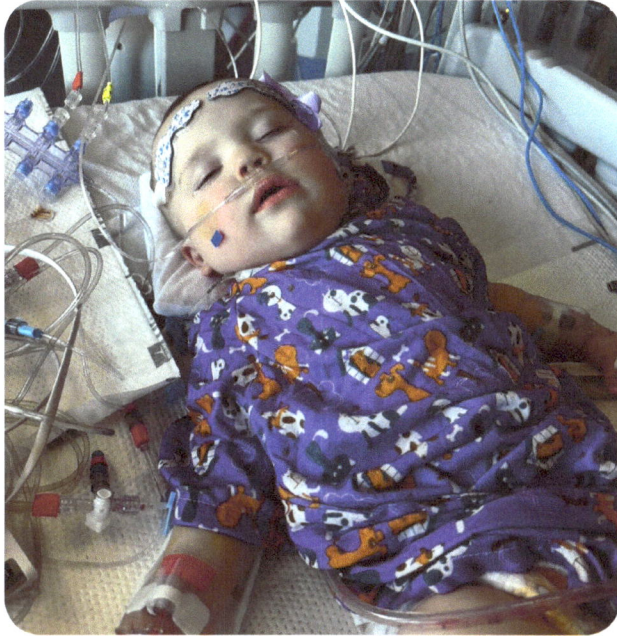
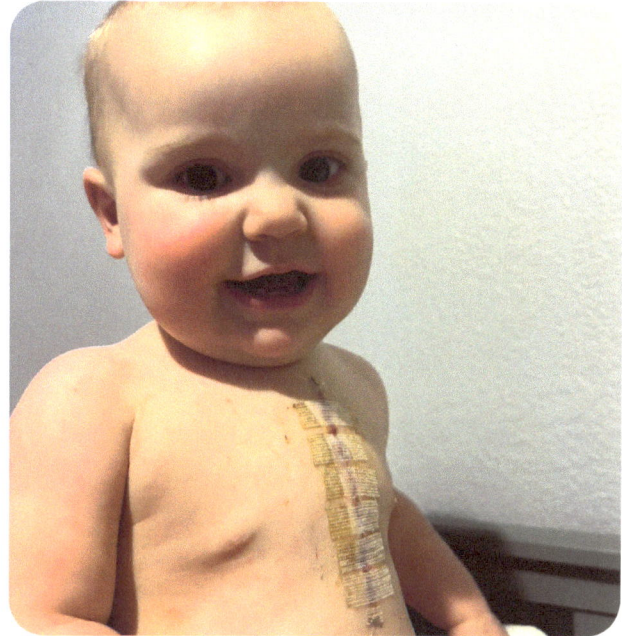
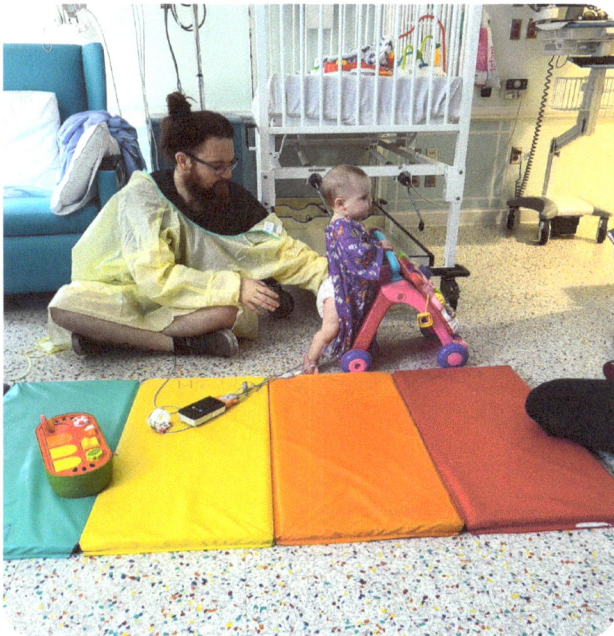
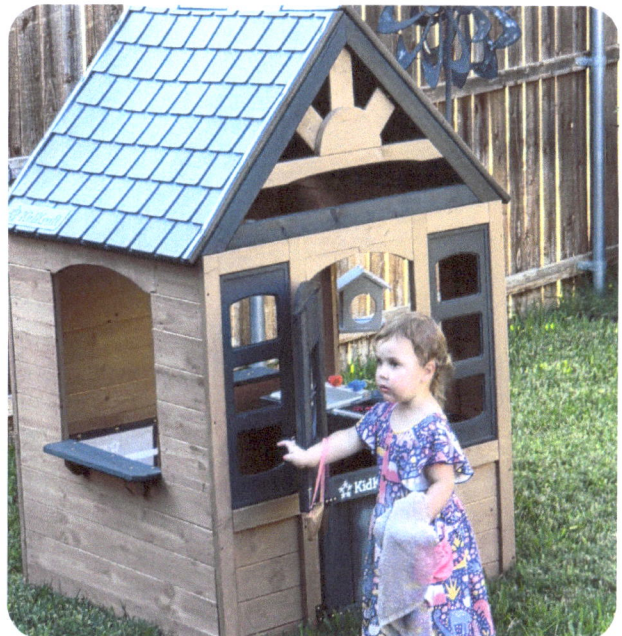

www.ingramcontent.com/pod-product-compliance
Lightning Source LLC
Chambersburg PA
CBHW060900270326
41935CB00003B/46

9781963514247